C. Diff In 30 Minutes

A Guide To Clostridium Difficile For Patients And Families

By J. Thomas Lamont, M.D.

Table Of Contents

Foreword

Welcome to *C. diff In 30 Minutes*. If you or a family member have been diagnosed with C. diff, you're dealing with diarrhea and other nasty symptoms, not to mention a decreased quality of life and worries about what comes next. This guide is intended to help explain what comes next, by answering basic questions about the C. diff bacteria and how it impacts the lives of victims, family members, and caregivers. It is also intended to reassure. While some patients despair that they will never recover, there are in fact a range of treatment options that not only offer relief, but actually lead to a cure. Of course, any treatment of C. diff must be made after discussions with your doctor.

The author of *C. Diff In 30 Minutes* is Gastroenterologist and Harvard Medical School Professor Dr. J. Thomas Lamont. Over the past three decades, Dr. Lamont has treated thousands of patients suffering from C. diff and has conducted ground-breaking research on the bacterium and its associated toxins. Using plain English, he will explain the basics of C. diff, ranging from causes to treatments. He will also explore more specific topics, such as:

- How C. diff impacts the daily lives of people suffering an infection

- Why family members and health-care providers are unlikely to catch C. diff from sick patients

- Dealing with recurring bouts of C. diff

- Antibiotics used to treat C. diff, as well as costs and recurrence rates

- Best practices for preventing the spread of C. diff

- Cutting-edge treatments, such as stool replacement

- Why a recurrence is more likely for adults aged 60 or over

- How some people become carriers of C. diff — but don't suffer any symptoms of the disease

- When it's safe to give the "all clear" signal.

The author also describes four cases involving C. diff infections. Through the stories of a new mother, an electrician, a grandmother, and a schoolteacher, you'll learn how C. diff impacts the lives of ordinary people, the types of treatment that are available, and what the road to recovery looks like.

C. Diff In 30 Minutes also includes a glossary of terms and medications, located at the back of the guide and online at cdiff.in30minutes.com. The companion web site also contains additional resources, such as an online glossary, videos, and other information of use to C. diff patients.

Introduction

Clostridium difficile — commonly referred to as "C. diff" — is a serious bacterial infection of the colon (large bowel). C. diff was first recognized in the 1970s. Since that initial discovery, C. diff has exploded, with more and more cases reported every year in North America, Europe, and further afield. In the past five years, C. diff has spread across the globe, helped in large part by air travel, the availability and frequent use of antibiotics, and the graying of the world's population.

Hospitals in almost every country have reported outbreaks of C. diff, and the number and severity of cases continues to soar. In 2010 there were 350,000 cases of C. diff diagnosed in U.S. hospitals. That means that of 1,000 patients admitted to U.S hospitals, 10 will become infected with C. diff, most of them elderly. In some hospitals and nursing homes, as many as one in five patients is infected.

C. diff Hospital Stays in the U.S. (in thousands)

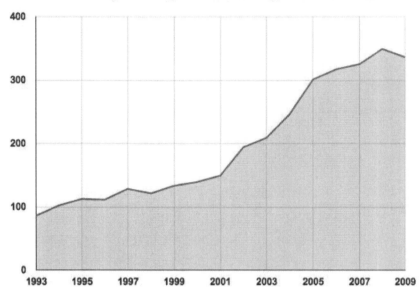

Source: Agency for Healthcare Research and Quality

Many people infected with C. diff are sick with diarrhea, abdominal pain, nausea, and weight loss. Others are "carriers" of C. diff with no signs or symptoms of disease. Some of these carriers have been recently infected with C. diff but have recovered and now feel well. But carriers still have the C. diff organism in their stools and can serve as a silent reservoir of infection in hospitals and nursing homes.

The purpose of this guide is to provide patients and their families with basic information and practical advice about C. diff infection. The number of chronic infections is rising yearly, and many patients (and sometimes their doctors) aren't sure what to do next. C. diff is not a simple "stomach bug" like viral gastroenteritis or food poisoning that disappears in nearly all patients after a week or two. As we discuss in Chapter 3, C. diff can be cured initially by one of these antibiotics:

- Metronidazole (sold under the commercial name Flagyl in the United States)

- Vancomycin (also called Vanco)

- Fidaxomycin (sold as Dificid in the United States)

Unfortunately for many patients, that is not the end of the story. A serious problem is the recurrence rate of 15-30%, much higher than we see in any other infection. Some patients suffer multiple recurrences over months or even years. This book is written especially for patients who can't seem to shake their C. diff, and who get sick with diarrhea again and again.

The situation is not hopeless, though. Even if you have a long-term C. diff infection, you can be helped and eventually cured. The more you understand about your infection, the better you will be able to start on the road to recovery.

Chapter 1:

Patient Stories: The Many Faces Of C. Diff

Like most diseases, C. diff infection comes in many forms, from mild to moderate, from severe to fatal. The infection is grouped into three levels of duration:

Type	Duration
Acute	1-3 weeks
Sub-acute	4-8 weeks
Chronic	Months to years

A very small number of patients will carry the infection for the rest of their lives, but they will have no symptoms and will not die from it. Some patients with C. diff do not need to be hospitalized and can be treated successfully as outpatients. Others, probably the majority, are in the hospital when they get the infection. The sickest patients among those will need to be treated in an intensive care unit (ICU). Among frail, elderly patients, C. diff can be fatal in approximately 5-10%. Some patients with severe C. diff end up losing their colon and have a permanent bag on their side to catch bodily waste, via a procedure known as an ileostomy.

Below are four C. diff case histories. Their names, identities, and other details have been changed to protect their privacy, and the photos are not of real patients. You, a friend or a family member may have experiences similar to Jeannie, Al, Mrs. E, and Martina. While these patients are quite different, they share a few things in common: All were healthy and active before they got C. diff, but eventually felt that the infection had taken over their lives. Even though the infection severely impacted their lives and caused worry for them and their family members, the good news is that all eventually recovered and have returned to their original health status.

Jeannie's Story: "My stomach feels terrible"

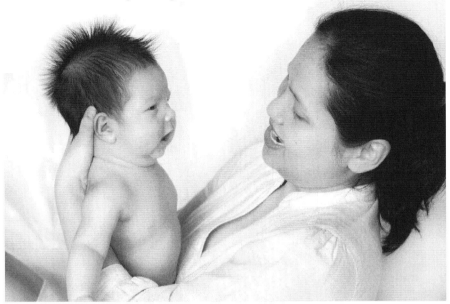

When I first visited Jeannie in her hospital bed in our obstetric service, she had delivered her firstborn, a healthy 7-pound, 8-ounce boy, six days earlier. Her pregnancy was uneventful, but after she was in labor for 36 hours her obstetrician decided that it was time for a C-section. The surgery was uneventful. However, four days later, Jeannie spiked a fever of 101 degrees from an infection in her incision. Her doctor ordered that she begin taking the antibiotic Ciprofloxacin by vein. After a few doses, the fever dropped and the incision looked better, with less redness and tenderness. At that point, Jeannie was anxious to go home with her new baby.

On the evening prior to discharge, she suddenly took a turn for the worse. Jeannie felt nauseated after supper, and complained of cramps in her left lower abdomen. Her condition quickly deteriorated. She was nauseated and vomiting, and she was passing watery diarrhea every hour. By midnight, she was passing watery stools every 20 or 30 minutes. The night resident examined her and decided that Jeannie probably had viral food poisoning from Norovirus. At the time, an outbreak of this common infection was going through the hospital, causing acute vomiting and diarrhea in patients and staff. The resident ordered stool tests and blood work, and told the nursing staff to increase her IV fluids and to hold all food. An injection was given to ease the nausea.

Jeannie felt a bit better for a few hours and dozed off. But by 5 a.m. the diarrhea was worse. Her pulse began to climb, and her blood pressure fell, tell-tale signs that she was getting dehydrated. The nurses noted that Jeannie was tearful and confused. She was unable to control her bowel movements and too sick to get out of bed to use the bathroom. The OB resident was concerned too, and Jeannie was quickly transferred to the ICU with a diagnosis of acute infection of the colon with severe dehydration.

The next morning Jeannie was very ill. Her skin was flushed and hot, and her tongue was dry. She could barely answer questions and was clearly confused. She couldn't remember much about what happened overnight and kept repeating, "My stomach feels terrible." Her belly was swollen and very tender to touch. When we listened with a stethoscope, her bowel was quiet. The room smelled of diarrhea, which had soiled her gown and bed.

At that point Jeannie's diagnosis was fulminant C. diff colitis with toxic megacolon. Let's break down what this means:

- **Fulminant** – severe, and quickly getting worse. See Chapter 3 for an explanation of Fulminant C. diff

- **C. diff colitis** – Colitis is inflammation, or swelling, of the colon. C.

diff is always concentrated in the colon or large bowel.

- **Megacolon** – Greatly dilated lower bowel caused by infections including C. diff.

In other words, Jeannie was facing a severe infection that had created a massive enlargement of her colon. It was a life-threatening condition. Within a few hours the laboratory reported that her stool from the night before tested positive for C. diff.

Because some patients with C. diff and toxic megacolon are so sick that they require a colectomy (surgical removal of the colon), we immediately called the surgery team to examine her. The surgeons didn't think she needed an emergency colectomy and advised medical management with antibiotics. We treated Jeannie with two antibiotics, metronidazole (sold as Flagyl in the United States) given by vein and vancomycin (sold as Vanco) by mouth. Over the next few days she gradually improved, and within a week she was discharged. When I saw her in the office a few weeks later, she was much better and ready to focus on her new baby. Jeannie gradually completely recovered. Two years after the initial infection, her bowel function was completely normal.

Takeaways

Jeannie's case illustrates several important points:

- C. diff can sometimes be life-threatening, even in healthy young adults.

- In certain cases, doctors have to consider a colectomy to save the patient's life.

- Once a patient gets rid of C. diff, bowel function returns to normal, and recovery is generally complete.

However, as we'll see in the next case, not everyone has such a straightforward recovery from a C. diff infection.

Al's Story: "My C. diff won't go away"

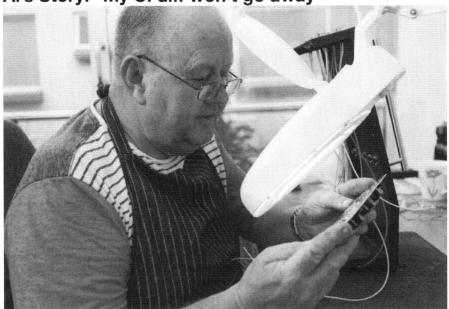

Al was a very healthy 62-year-old electrician. That is, until he developed an abscess on his wisdom tooth. His dentist prescribed the antibiotic clindamycin for seven days to treat the abscess and scheduled a root canal.

Five days after Al finished the clindamycin, he developed diarrhea, an upset stomach, and pain in the lower abdomen. The diarrhea was severe, occurring up to 10 times per day. He called his doctor who tested his stools for C. diff. The result was positive. Treatment was started with 10 days of Flagyl (one of the same antibiotics taken by Jeannie) four times per day. By the fifth day, his diarrhea was almost gone and Al was ready to go back to work.

Four days later the diarrhea returned. It was as bad as it had been in the beginning. This time, Al's doctor started him on Vanco (the other antibiotic taken by Jeannie) four times per day. Again, Al appeared to recover, and the diarrhea went away. But eight days after Al stopped the Vanco, it came back — the same smelly diarrhea with lots of mucus and cramps. Al was frustrated now and worried that he might never get rid of his C. diff.

His primary care doctor was frustrated, too. He arranged for Al to see an infectious disease specialist at a teaching hospital in Boston. The specialist recommended a pulse-taper of vancomycin for eight weeks, during which the Vanco was taken in a gradually decreasing dose. It started with one capsule four times per day, and ended with one capsule every other day for the last week. Al finished the eight weeks of Vanco and followed this up with four weeks of Culturelle, a probiotic. Probiotics are dried bacteria or yeasts that are designed to help the colonic flora, the bacteria and other microorganisms that live in our large bowel (colon), to return to their original state before the patient took antibiotic treatment.

This time, the diarrhea came back two weeks after he stopped taking Vanco. Al's frustration level went through the roof. He felt that C. diff had taken over his life and he would never get better. He even worried that his C. diff infection was going to be fatal. At that point, his son went online to see what options were available for patients with multiple recurrences of C. diff. He read that many patients like his father got better after a **stool transplant**.

Getting a stool transplant is like reseeding a lawn that has been damaged by weeds, drought, and poor soil. The soil is prepared, watered, and seeded, and eventually a new lawn replaces the old. In a stool transplant, the "seeds" are a suspension or "shake" of healthy stool, taken from a healthy donor, and transferred via a medical device to the colon of a person suffering from C. diff. The procedure is straightforward and has a permanent cure rate of 95% among C. diff patients. Chapter 3 describes the procedure in more detail.

Al was eventually referred to a gastroenterologist (GI) specialist at our hospital who had experience with stool transplants to treat C. diff. The doctor explained that the C. diff infection kept coming back because Al's colonic flora was depleted from all the antibiotics taken over the past three months. The normal colonic flora provides a protective barrier against C. diff, other harmful bacteria, and viruses. That's why nearly every patient who gets C. diff has taken an antibiotic before the diarrhea starts. But Al's barrier was so low that the C. diff kept coming back after he stopped the Vanco.

Once patients have had one recurrence, the odds go way up that they will have multiple repeat attacks. We have seen patients with more than 10 such recurrences. They are typically elderly with other illnesses such as heart failure, cancer, or chronic kidney disease, all of which can depress the immune system. Depression, fatigue, and weight loss are very common in so-called "repeaters."

In order to try a stool transplant, a donor was needed. Al's wife was healthy, with no diarrhea and no recent antibiotics. The plan was for her to come in with Al on the day of his colonoscopy, and to "donate" a stool sample that would be used to reseed his colon. Her stool was put in a blender with water to make a thin liquid shake, which was then filtered to remove any solid material. The GI doctor then passed a colonoscope to the upper part of Al's colon and injected some of his wife's liquefied stool through the scope. Then he slowly withdrew the scope, infusing some of the liquid every four or five inches until he reached the bottom of the colon. Al was instructed to lie quietly for an hour in the recovery area, and then he was discharged home with instructions to take no more vancomycin.

After the transplant Al felt fine. Naturally, he worried that C. diff might come back. When he saw the gastrointestinal doctor three weeks later, he had no diarrhea, the longest time he had been without symptoms since the root canal. Three months after the stool transplant, Al was feeling great and working full time. He was cured!

At our hospital we have performed dozens of stool transplants for patients with recurrent C. diff. All but one were completely successful, and the one patient who failed had a second attempt that was eventually successful.

For C. diff patients who have tried everything, stool transplants can make a huge difference. Some patients are afraid to try a stool transplant because it seems "gross" or "yucky." But in hundreds if not thousands of patients worldwide the procedure is safe and very effective. The source of the stool is usually a family member or friend. For a lot of our patients who have recurring C. diff, the choice is either a transplant or more antibiotics for a long time.

Takeaways

Al's case also illustrates several aspects of recurrent C. diff, a huge problem that occurs in up to 30% of patients who get C. diff after the initial treatment with the antibiotics Flagyl or Vanco.

- In these unfortunate cases, the infection comes back or recurs within days or weeks of stopping the antibiotics.

- Some unlucky patients experience ten or more recurrences and start to think they will never recover.

- Al got C. diff in the "community," not in a hospital, like most patients.

- The antibiotic, clindamycin, that he received to treat his dental abscess, set him up for the C. diff by wiping out his good colonic bacteria allowing the C. diff to get in.

Community-acquired C. diff is much more common in the last five years. This means that the organism is now more widespread in the general population. Where Al got his infection after he took the clindamycin remains a mystery. He wasn't in contact with any patients with known C. diff, and hadn't visited a hospital or nursing home. Some studies have reported C. diff in food purchased in a supermarket. Dogs, horses, pigs, and rabbits can also be carriers of C. diff, although spread of disease from pets or domestic animals to humans has yet to be documented. Like most infections, it is usually impossible to pinpoint the source of C. diff.

Mrs. E: "Do you think I will ever be rid of this awful C. diff?"

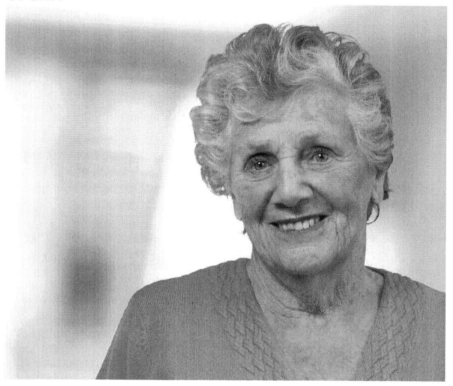

Mrs. E was a feisty 80-year-old grandmother living alone in her home with two cats and a canary. She came to my office because she wasn't sure her C. diff was gone.

Her story started three months earlier, after she had a knee replacement. During her recovery, she developed a fever and received the antibiotic Cipro for just three days. A week after discharge, she got a C. diff infection while staying in a rehab hospital. After a week of diarrhea, her doctor tested her stool for C. diff. When the test came back positive, she was started on Flagyl, the same antibiotic taken by both Jeannie and Al. Her response was excellent, and five days later she was no longer having any diarrhea.

After Mrs. E had finished the Flagyl and was back home again, she visited her doctor who decided to test her stool for C. diff to see if it was gone. To his surprise and to Mrs. E's disappointment, the test came back positive. A second course of Flagyl was started, even though she was feeling fine. A few weeks after that, her stool again tested positive. After several more courses of Flagyl, which had no effect on her stool test, she came to see me for a second opinion. Her first words in the office were "Do you think I will ever be rid of this awful C. diff?"

In fact, it was easy to reassure Mrs. E that she did not need any more stool tests to see if she still had C. diff, and she definitely didn't need any more Flagyl. And yes, she would eventually get rid of the C. diff. She just needed to be patient and wait for her normal colonic flora to recover, a process that can take one to three months after the last dose of antibiotic.

Mrs. E's story is very common, and it's one that can be confusing to patients and their doctors. Her case is an example of the **post-convalescent C. diff carrier state**. This occurs when patients recover from diarrhea and other C. diff symptoms, usually in the first week of treatment, However it may take months before the C. diff finally disappears from the stool. During this time the patient is passing C. diff in the stool, which can infect other people. Carriers have no diarrhea or other symptoms because they have developed antibodies to the C. diff toxins. These antibodies neutralize the toxins and prevent diarrhea, fever, and cramps. But the C. diff lingers in the bowel. How? It takes advantage of the lowered resistance of the colonic flora caused by the original antibiotic. In Mrs. E's case the antibiotic Cipro was used to treat her knee infection, and Flagyl was used to treat her C. diff.

We'll cover the importance of healthy colonic flora later in the guide, but for the time being, understand that Mrs. E was in a sort of limbo, in which the symptoms of the disease are gone (no diarrhea, pain or fever) but the C. diff lingers for a while (stool test still positive). More information about convalescent carriers can be found in Chapter 2.

Takeaways

Mrs. E's case illustrates several important points:

- Once the diarrhea and other symptoms of C. diff are gone and their antibiotic treatments are finished (usually within 10 days), we don't recommend testing the stool for C. diff. In most infections, including bowel infections, strep throat and even colds and the flu, patients can be shedding the causative organism long after the symptoms have resolved.

- Testing stools for C. diff in patients after they have finished their Flagyl or Vanco for 10 days and after their bowel movements have returned to normal (that is, formed and not watery) is a waste of time and money, and is not helpful to the doctor or patient.

- Even if the stool test is positive, treatment is not required. In fact, re-treatment of stool carriers doesn't work, as more antibiotic therapy prolongs the carrier state. The goal is to allow the colonic flora to recover, something that can't happen if more antibiotics are given.

Once the colonic flora is back to baseline, C. diff will be gone for good. Stated simply: Patience is required, not more antibiotics.

Martina's Story: "My C. diff is gone, so why do I still have diarrhea?"

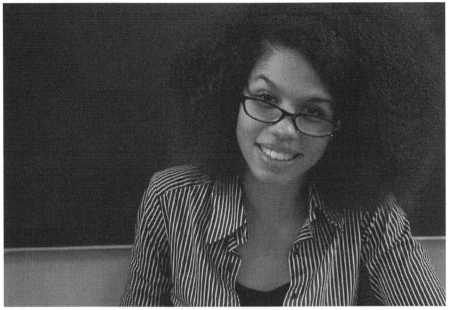

Martina, a schoolteacher in a suburb of Boston, got C. diff when she was hospitalized for pneumonia. First, she caught a cold from one of her fifth-graders. A few days later, she spiked a fever, and felt short of breath. A chest x-ray in the emergency room showed right lower-lobe pneumonia. She was admitted to the hospital for three days and quickly responded to treatment with Levaquin (levofloxacin), a strong antibiotic used to treat pneumonia and other infections.

C. diff diarrhea started a week after she was discharged. The infection responded quickly to a 10-day course of Vanco. She felt well, except for one or two loose stools in the morning, with gas and bloating. A month after she had pneumonia, her stools were still not back to normal, so she asked her doctor if she could be tested again for C. diff. A stool test for C. diff was

25

negative, but Martina was still worried that her infection was back.

Over the next few weeks her diarrhea increased to three or four mushy or watery stools daily, with more gas and bloating. She gave up spicy foods and coffee, and went on a lactose-free diet. None of these actions helped very much.

To make matters worse, the diarrhea was coming on without much warning, so she felt she had to stay close to the bathroom, especially in the morning. One day she had a near accident in her classroom, barely making it to the bathroom. That's when Martina decided she needed another opinion.

By the time she was seen, Martina was a nervous wreck. "I must have C. diff again with all this diarrhea," she told the doctor. But a repeat stool test for C. diff was again negative, and a colonoscopy and biopsies showed nothing abnormal. Blood tests for other conditions that might explain her symptoms — celiac disease (gluten-sensitive enteropathy) and overactive thyroid — were negative.

Martina was diagnosed with **post-infectious irritable bowel syndrome (IBS)**, a type of diarrhea that can follow a bowel infection like C. diff or salmonella food poisoning. For reasons that are unclear, women are much more susceptible to IBS than men. This condition results from damage or irritation to the lining of the bowel and to the muscles and nerves that regulate bowel function. It is more likely to occur in patients who had a diagnosis of IBS in the past.

Martina was treated with Imodium, an over-the-counter anti-diarrheal pill. She needed a lot of reassurance that her C. diff was gone and that she didn't have some other serious bowel problem. Doctors are seeing increasing numbers of patients with IBS after C. diff, some of whom complain of severe diarrhea that is almost as bad as the original infection. It's important in these patients for the doctor to rule out recurrent C. diff or other causes of diarrhea such as ulcerative colitis, Crohn's disease, celiac disease, or overactive thyroid.

Martina's diarrhea gradually diminished, and six months later her bowel movements were back to baseline.

I tell my patients with post-infectious IBS that the diarrhea and other symptoms are usually gone in six to twelve months. Emphasizing that they do not have active C. diff infection is also very reassuring.

Takeaways:

There are several takeaways from Martina's case:

- Not every patient with diarrhea after treatment for C. diff has recurrent infection.

- Make sure it's not IBS, celiac disease, lactose intolerance, or overactive thyroid, which can start after a bowel infection.

- A negative stool test rules out C. diff.

Chapter 2:

C. Diff: A Nasty Bug With Bad Toxins

Clostridium difficile (also known as the "difficult Clostridium") got its unusual name when it was first described in 1935. The doctors who discovered it had a difficult time getting the bug to grow in the lab so they could study it.

At the time, C. diff wasn't known to cause any illness. In fact, it was found in the stools of healthy newborns where it is part of the normal colonic flora in the first year of life. Only in 1977 was C. diff identified as the cause of antibiotic-associated colitis. Now it is a serious problem in hospitals and nursing homes around the world. What follows are some facts and figures about this nasty bug and how it causes such bad diarrhea.

C. diff produces two toxins, called toxin A and toxin B. These toxins cause the diarrhea and colitis. Bacterial toxins are like smart bombs that seek and destroy their target. C. diff toxins are released into the bowel where they attach to the lining cells and trigger severe diarrhea and inflammation. C. diff and its toxins also are excreted into the stool where they can be identified in the clinical laboratory. Testing a stool for the presence of the toxins or the bug itself is how we diagnose a C. diff infection.

Once the infection is treated with 10 days of Flagyl or Vanco, C. diff gradually disappears from the stool over a two- to three-month period as the normal flora comes back. However, some patients experience a recurrence, a condition which is described in Chapter 3.

Convalescent Carriers

As we discussed earlier in Mrs. E's case, carriers are patients who have been treated for C. diff infection but still have the organism and its toxins in their stool even though they do not have diarrhea or other symptoms. These individuals are called "convalescent carriers," which means that the C. diff is still living in the colon but the symptoms are gone. C. diff gradually diminishes in number and then disappears for good. This sequence of events occurs in the majority of patients (70-80%). Later we will discuss what happens to the other 20-30% of patients who experience a recurrence.

How C. Diff Spreads

C. diff is a contagious disease. However, it usually doesn't spread directly from one person to another like influenza, strep throat or common colds. Patients pick up C. diff from the environment, typically a hospital or nursing home.

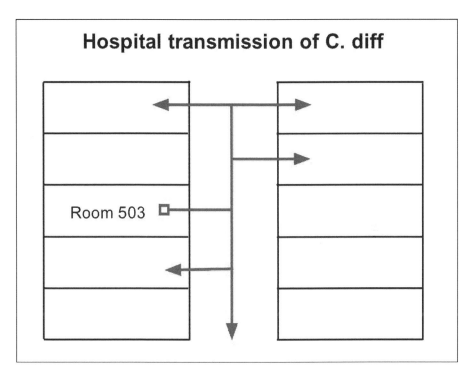

Hospital transmission of C. diff

Room 503

Here's how it happens. Let's imagine a C. diff patient, Mrs. Smith, in Room 503, in our hospital. She has acute C. diff infection and is passing liquid stools (diarrhea) 10 times per day. Billions of C. diff organisms are in her stools. Tiny amounts of the C. diff organisms get on the sheets, linen, toilet seat, telephone, and floor in her room. When doctors come in to examine Mrs. Smith, they may pick up C. diff spores on their hands, clothing, or stethoscopes. Depending on how well they wash their hands and clean their stethoscopes, C. diff can hitch a ride to the next patient they examine and infect that patient ... especially if that patient is taking an antibiotic.

Once C. diff leaves the colon of the infected patient in a liquid stool, it usually converts to a spore that is like a seed that lies dormant in the hospital until it gets picked up by a suitable human host. Once swallowed,

C. diff germinates (hatches) in the bowel and starts a new cycle of infection.

Since the spores of C. diff are able to survive for months or even years in the hospital environment, it's possible that spores from one patient can infect another patient admitted to the same hospital room even months later. It is almost impossible to know with certainty how or where a given patient picks up C. diff, because the spores are so common in the hospital environment. Spores of C. diff can be found in soil, in the home, and even in the supermarket. Patients pick them up on their hands and transfer them to their mouth when they eat.

Note, however, that airborne transmission is unlikely for a stomach infection, as airborne particles end up in the lungs (like the common cold, which can be transmitted by a sneeze). C. diff germinates in the bowel.

Person-to-person transmission is also rare. It's extremely unlikely for a husband with a C. diff infection to pass it to his wife, or for a parent to pass it to his child, unless the wife or the child is taking an antibiotic.

However, spread from one patient to another in the same hospital room can occur. Because of this, patients diagnosed with C. diff are usually moved to a private room. When patients with C. diff are discharged from the hospital, their room and furniture are cleaned thoroughly with bleach to kill C. diff to prevent the next patient from getting infected. Doctors are required to clean their hands with hand sanitizer or soap and water before and after examining a patient. When this rule is strictly enforced, it reduces the rate of C. diff infection in hospitals and nursing homes.

Limiting The Spread Of C. Diff

Patients are often terrified that they will spread the infection to family or friends. As noted earlier in this chapter, this is extremely rare.

Consider that doctors examining C. diff patients in their office do not wear gowns, gloves, or masks. In fact, doctors examine thousands of C. diff-infected patients every year — but they are rarely infected. For friends and family members, the risk of infection is similarly unlikely.

C. diff is transmitted to patients by ingestion of spores from the environment. Only a small fraction of patients taking antibiotics (one in a hundred to one in a thousand) develop C. diff infection, so the risk of transmission to anyone is very small. The risk of transmitting C. diff to a personal contact who is not taking antibiotics is even smaller. At our hospital, we recommend the following measures to prevent the spread of C. diff:

Doctors and nurses: Hand washing with soap and water, or with alcohol-based hand sanitizers, before and after examining patients with C. diff.

Patients with C. diff: Wash your hands thoroughly with soap and warm water for one minute after using the bathroom, and wipe down the toilet seat with alcohol wipes if you are passing liquid stool.

Family members: Wash you hands with soap and water before eating to avoid ingesting C. diff spores, especially if you are taking an antibiotic.

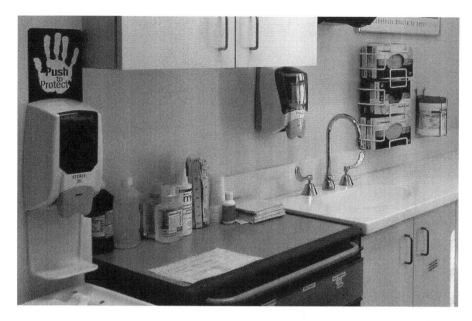

Spores are incredibly durable and can survive for years. While hand washing with soap kills C. diff spores, hand sanitizers do not. However, because hand sanitizers are convenient and portable, and don't require a sink or hot water, they are a reasonable second-line recommendation.

Why Do Some Patients Get C. Diff After Taking Antibiotics?

To get C. diff infection two things have to happen:

1. The patient takes an antibiotic that weakens the protective organisms that normally live in the bowel.

2. The patient swallows some spores of C. diff.

Certainly not everyone who takes an antibiotic gets C. diff. Likewise, not everyone who swallows a spore will become infected. But these two factors are thought to be necessary for disease transmission.

The Importance Of A Healthy Colon

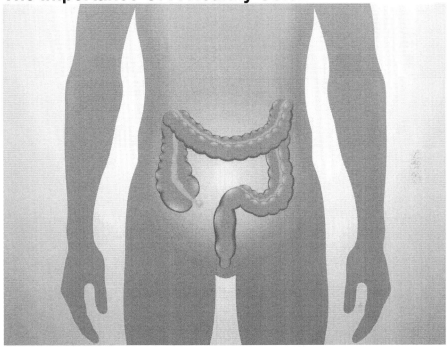

Although it may seem unlikely, the stool in your colon serves a very important function. That's right, the smelly stuff you flush down the toilet is actually extremely important to your overall health and well-being. Your colon (highlighted in the above image) is loaded with trillions of microorganisms, including bacteria, viruses, and fungi, which live there in perfect harmony with each other and with you. In fact, these tiny organisms count on you to feed and water them every day, just like your pet cat or dog.

About 90% of the food you eat is absorbed by your intestinal tract. Every cell in your body, from the hair on your head to the skin on the soles of your feet, is made from the food you eat.

What about the rest? The 10% that's not absorbed feeds the trillions of bowel flora living in your colon. Ten percent of your diet is mostly plant fibers, cereals, and starches, sometimes called roughage, which cannot be digested and absorbed by humans. For centuries, scientists had little knowledge about the colonic flora, but now it's clear that the organisms in our stools protect us from invaders like C. diff and other causes of bowel infection. These bacteria in the colon are sometimes called "the barrier flora" because they provide a protective shield against harmful organisms. The image below shows a type of barrier flora, magnified by an electron microscope.

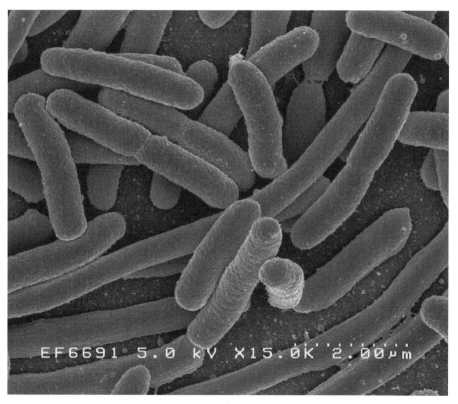

Antibiotics can have a negative impact on the flora in your colon. While antibiotics are used to treat bacterial infections, such as strep throat or tuberculosis, they can also take out the barrier flora and other normal bacteria in your colon.

So, to get C. diff, the first thing that has to happen is that your barrier flora are killed off or weakened by an antibiotic. Once this happens, C. diff can jump in. Clearly this doesn't happen to everyone who takes an antibiotic. Only about 1 in 100 or 1 in 1,000 people who take an antibiotic will get C. diff. Not all antibiotics are equal in their ability to allow C. diff. Clindamycin, ciprofloxacin, penicillins and cephalosporins are the main offenders, while azithromycin, tetracycline and bactrim are less likely to cause this problem.

The bottom line: Any antibiotic can weaken your barrier flora in the bowel that normally protects you from invasion by C. diff.

C. Diff In Infants: An Unsolved Mystery

C. diff was originally discovered in healthy babies, who seem to tolerate this nasty bug in their stools without getting sick. About 70% of infants during the first year of life carry C. diff. Why they don't show signs of disease like diarrhea or fever remains a mystery.

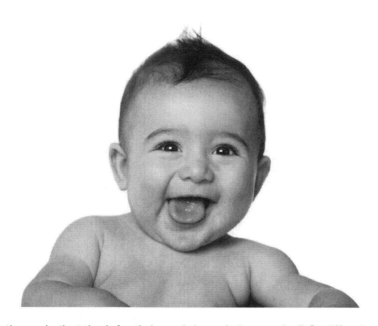

One theory is that the infant's bowel doesn't "recognize" C. diff or its toxins. C. diff toxins cause diarrhea by hooking on to a special toxin receptor, much like a key opens a lock. Once the toxin (the key) hooks on to its receptor (the lock), it opens the floodgates of diarrhea and causes fever, cramps, and other signs of acute infection. Healthy infants lack this receptor, so they don't get sick even though they are carrying enough C. diff to cause severe diarrhea in an adult. After the first year of life, babies develop the receptor and can develop C. diff just like adults. So, finding C. diff in the stool of an infant is not worrisome. Eventually, C. diff will disappear from the intestinal tract when the infant reaches 10-12 months.

Can babies spread C. diff to other family members, babysitters, or health-care workers? The answer is yes, but in practice it's very rare. Sometimes mothers of newborn babies have to take antibiotics for a urinary tract infection. The antibiotics can damage the protective stool barrier allowing C.

diff to get in and cause infection. I have treated a few moms who probably caught C. diff from their newborns. I have also treated a neonatologist (a pediatric specialist in newborn diseases) who probably picked up C. diff at work from one of her sick newborns.

Even though babies can carry C. diff, we don't recommend any special precautions to mothers or other family members. Catching C. diff from a baby is so rare that enforcing special precautions is probably not necessary. Wearing rubber gloves when diapering, or hand washing after changing diapers, is always recommended, especially if the person changing the diaper is taking an antibiotic.

Being a carrier of C. diff is beneficial to the baby. Healthy babies who are carriers develop an immune reaction to C. diff toxins that results in the formation of antibodies that protect against C. diff infection. Immunity to C. diff developing during the first year of life can last a lifetime and protect patients who later come in contact with C. diff. Those who have antibodies become "carriers" with no diarrhea, while those with no antibody can develop full-blown C. diff. Since about 70% of babies are carriers, this implies that they will likely never get C. diff in their lifetimes!

How your Immune System Fights C. Diff

Infections of any kind usually stimulate your immune system to make antibodies, special proteins produced by immune cells that live in your spleen, lymph nodes, and other organs including the bowel. Antibodies protect you by binding to bacteria or bacterial toxins and neutralizing them so they are harmless. Antibodies can result either from an infection, or by a vaccination. As noted earlier, about 70% of healthy infants carry C. diff and its toxins. Such "infantile carriers" form antibodies to C. diff, which are protective for life. Patients who get C. diff infection in childhood or adulthood also form antibodies that protect against a second infection. Like infection with mumps or measles, patients with C. diff generally do not get a second C. diff infection years later.

However, there are exceptions. Patients with recurrent disease have many bouts of C. diff, but these patients fail to generate antibodies (this is discussed below). Other patients may generate antibodies after infection but may lose the protection later on if their immune system is weakened by diseases, drugs, or old age. Bottom line: A healthy immune system and a healthy colonic flora are needed to protect against C. diff infection.

As for what foods should be eaten to help colonic flora, it's hard to tell. Consider the fact that people from China, Mexico, Egypt, and the United States typically have different things for breakfast, lunch, and dinner. No matter what they eat, they all seem to have barrier flora. It's not necessarily the food we eat, but rather the germs on that food that seed our bowel.

Why Does C. Diff Sometimes Keep Coming Back?

After initial "cure" of C. diff with antibiotics, about 15-25% develop a recurrence within a few days to several months. The chance of a recurrence depends in large part on the type of antibiotic being taken, such as Flagyl, Vanco, or Dificid, as well as the age of the patient.

This repeat infection can keep on recurring, even after multiple courses of antibiotics. We have seen some unfortunate patients with 10 or more attacks of C. diff in a two-year period, causing chronic diarrhea, weight loss, and diminished quality of life.

We think that recurrence of C. diff depends on a "Perfect Storm" of several factors, including:

- Simultaneous failure of the immune system with inadequate antibody formation

- Failure of the colonic flora to regenerate, owing to exposure to antibiotics.

Failure of the immune system to generate an antibody response is quite common after age 60. The older the patient, the weaker the response to an infection or to vaccination. During an initial bout of C. diff infection, a healthy immune system develops antibodies that protect against another bout of C. diff infection. But after age 50 or so, this immune response is diminished. That's why recurrent C. diff infections are much more common in 80 year olds (35%) vs. 40 year olds (10%).

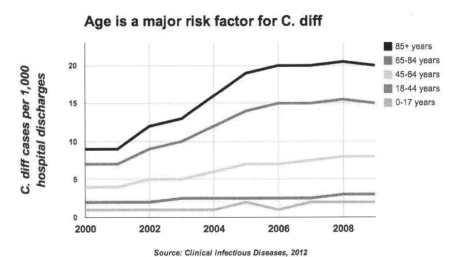

Age is a major risk factor for C. diff

Source: Clinical Infectious Diseases, 2012

Chapter 3:

Treatment Options For C. Diff Infection

C. diff treatment requires antibiotics available only by prescription, so the information below is not a do-it-yourself guide. It's provided to help you understand what your doctor is recommending and why.

In addition, just as not all doctors are trained or experienced enough to deliver a baby or treat a heart attack, some doctors are more likely than others to have the knowledge and experience to manage C. diff infections.

Generally, the first attack of C. diff is treated by the following types of doctors:

- Hospital doctors (hospitalists) with training in medicine, surgery, or obstetrics-gynecology (OB-GYN)

- Primary care physicians (PCP), pediatricians, or specialists in infectious diseases (ID) and gastroenterology (GI). Patients usually see these doctors in their offices or private practices.

Sometimes patients can't seem to connect with an experienced doctor who knows how to treat complicated C. diff. If you are having trouble finding a medical specialist with expertise in C. diff, try checking online databases of doctors that are maintained by health insurance companies. Look for gastroenterology and infectious disease specialists, who are generally familiar with C. diff or can recommend doctors who have experience treating the disease.

Treatment Of Acute C. Diff: The First Attack

Antibiotics are almost always involved in causing C. diff. Paradoxically, antibiotics are also the main treatment.

C. diff specialists divide antibiotics into two groups. The antibiotic that precedes this infection and weakens the colonic flora is called the "Inciting Antibiotic." The antibiotics we use to eradicate C. diff are called the "Treating Antibiotics."

It's important to note that just because a patient gets C. diff after taking a certain antibiotic, that doesn't imply antibiotics are to be avoided in the future. Antibiotics are one of the marvels of modern medicine and are one of he main reasons why you are likely to live a lot longer than your grandparents or great-grandparents. Getting C. diff doesn't mean you can never take antibiotics again. But C. diff specialists say some antibiotics should be avoided in certain circumstances, as will be discussed in more detail.

Inciting Antibiotics

Certain types of antibiotics are known to incite C. diff in certain patients. Here's a chart that lists those antibiotics, as well as antibiotics that are less likely to lead to a C. diff infection:

Association of Antibiotics and C. diff

FREQUENT	OCCASIONAL	RARELY
Ampicillin	Bactrim	Aminoglycosides
Amoxicillin	Biaxin	Metronidazole
Cephalosporins (inc. Keflex)	Erythromycin	Rifaxamin
Cipro	Macrobid or Furadantin	Tetracyclines
Clindamycin	Other penicillins	Vancomycin
Levofloxin	Quinolones	
	Trimethopim	
	Zithromax	

In patients with active C. diff infection, we almost always stop the inciting antibiotic unless the patient needs to continue it. For example, if a patient develops C. diff while being treated with an antibiotic for a serious blood infection (septicemia) or lung infection (pneumonia), the inciting antibiotics cannot be stopped.

However, if the inciting antibiotics were given for a cold or an infection that is probably already cured, then the doctors can advise to stop the antibiotics.

Treating Antibiotics

The main "treating antibiotics" are Flagyl, Vanco, and Dificid, all of which have been extensively tested in patients with C. diff. Vanco and Dificid are equally effective, with initial response rates of 90-95%. However, the recurrence rate (second infection) with Dificid is 15% compared to 25% with Vanco. Flagyl is less effective than either Vanco or Dificid, and has a recurrence rate of about 25%. Flagyl also has more side effects including stomach upset, metallic taste, and more serious side effects of peripheral neuropathy and alcohol sensitivity in 1-2% of people taking the antibiotic.

But Flagyl has a significant advantage over the other treatments: Low cost. A 14-day supply of Flagyl costs about $25, vs. $800-$1200 for Vanco and up to $2,000 for Dificid. These are retail costs for patients without insurance or have insurance that doesn't cover Vanco or Dificid. C. diff patients who must take these drugs but have to pay full price out of pocket should consider purchasing them online from Canada, where these antibiotics are sometimes cheaper.

The following chart summarizes the differences between the three antibiotics:

Antibiotics to treat C. diff

Commercial Antibiotic	Initial Response Rate	Recurrence Rate	Retail Cost (14 days)
Flagyl (metronidazole)	85%	25%	$25
Vanco (vancomycin)	90-95%	25%	$800-$1,200
Dificid (fidaxomicin)	90-95%	15%	$2,000

Approximately 50% of first attacks are treated with Flagyl, using a dose of 250 mg or 500 mg three or four times daily for 10 to 14 days. The next most-popular choice is Vanco at 125 mg by mouth four times daily. Dificid treatment is the most expensive by far and may not be covered by insurance. Optimer Pharmaceuticals, the company that makes Dificid, has a patient assistance program that provides a discount to help patients cover the cost of this antibiotic. Get more information at (855) 841-4236 or online at www.optimerpharma.com. The standard dose is 200 mg twice daily for 10 days. All three antibiotics can be taken with food to reduce stomach irritation.

Flagyl, Vanco, or Dificid start to work after two or three days. In 50-90% of patients, diarrhea is improved or gone altogether by the end of the first week of treatment. Lack of response or continued diarrhea in a C. diff patient after five days of treatment with one of these antibiotics is cause for concern, especially if the patient is taking the drug on schedule.

If the patient is non-compliant (that is, not taking the medicine on schedule), then the treatment obviously won't be effective. To help the patient remember to take his medications, a pill container with separate pill compartments for each day of the week, a drug calendar, or a simple checklist for each dose can help keep the patient on schedule.

If a C. diff patient is taking Flagyl, Vanco, or Dificid on schedule, but is still having diarrhea and other symptoms, this should raise an alarm signal that something else is going on. Further evaluation of the patient may be required. One of the main reasons for failure of C. diff treatment is that the patient doesn't really have C. diff or has C. diff but also has an additional cause for diarrhea. Sorting this out requires more testing and perhaps a change of medication. In some patients with severe C. diff, the standard doses of antibiotics are insufficient. These patients generally need to be admitted to hospital (if they are not already in the hospital) for treatment with intravenous medications and close observation in an ICU.

Treating Severe C. Diff

Fulminant C. diff refers to the most severe form of acute C. diff. This is a serious complication and carries the risk of a prolonged hospital stay, surgery, or even death. Fulminant C. diff is much more common in frail, older patients with the following types of medical or surgical conditions:

- Cancer

- Transplantation

- Diabetes

- Kidney failure

- Stroke

- Failure of the immune system related to lymphoma, leukemia or chemotherapy

Treatment is initiated with high-dose, intravenous Flagyl and oral Vancomycin or Dificid. Patients are closely monitored, and those who fail to respond or get worse over two or three days may require surgery to remove part of the colon, a procedure known as a sub-total colectomy. Even this measure may be insufficient to stop the downward spiral, and death occurs in up to 30% of patients with fulminant C. diff depending on their age, physical status, and other medical conditions.

Recurrent C. Diff

As noted earlier, C. diff comes back in 25% of patients who have successfully recovered after a 10- to 14-day course of Flagyl or Vanco, and 15% of patients who have taken Dificid. Hardly any other common infection, other than malaria and tuberculosis, keeps returning after an apparent cure.

A recurrent C. diff infection is indicated by the return of smelly diarrhea, similar to what the patient noted during the first attack. Some patients complain of fever, cramps in the lower abdomen, nausea and vomiting, and fatigue. Generally, recurrence happens within a few weeks after finishing antibiotics, but sometimes it can be longer, even up to three months later.

How To Tell That C. Diff Has Returned

Patients can often tell that their C. diff is back because of its characteristic rancid and nauseating odor. Some of our hospital nurses can also "tell by the smell" that a patient has C. diff. This is not as crazy as it sounds. C. diff releases several volatile, fatty acids in the colon that are very malodorous (a medical term for "stinky"). The smell can be worse than even the stench of ordinary feces.

Treatment of recurrent C. diff is sometimes more complicated than treatment of a single bout of infection. When patients develop recurrent diarrhea after an initial bout of C. diff, the diagnosis of C. diff needs to be confirmed by a stool test for C. diff. The recent rapid stool tests for C. diff provide the result within eight-twelve hours. If that test returns positive, treatment is initiated with 14 days of either Flagyl or Vanco at the same dose as used for the first attack. If the diarrhea is severe (more than six times daily), or the patient complains of nausea, vomiting, cramps, or fever, Vanco or Dificid would be recommended over Flagyl, even if it was curative for the initial attack. This approach is successful in 40-50% of patients with a first recurrence.

Dealing With Second Recurrences And Beyond

Unfortunately, some 50-60% of patients who experience one recurrence get a second recurrence. After a second recurrence, about 80% of that group continue with recurrence after recurrence. Some unlucky patients may get 10 or more bouts. This is often accompanied by progressive weight loss, anxiety, depression, and seriously impaired quality of life. Patients are often convinced that the infection will never go away and that they will eventually die.

Management of recurrence is not as easy as treating a first attack. The medical literature does not provide exact guidelines as to the best way. Outlined below is what I do when patients have a second recurrence (that is, the third bout of diarrhea from C. diff).

Pulsed-Tapered Dosing Of Vanco

This approach is successful in getting rid of C. diff infection in about 50% of patients that have had a second recurrence. The idea is to extend the duration of the treatment by slowly tapering the dose over a three-month period. The details are shown in the table below.

Pulse-tapered Vanco treatment for recurrent C. difficile

Week 1	Vanco, 125 mg	Four times per day
Week 2	Vanco, 125 mg	Three times per day
Week 3	Vanco, 125 mg	Twice per day
Week 4	Vanco, 125 mg	Once per day
Week 5	Vanco, 125 mg	Once every other day
Week 6	Vanco, 125 mg	Once every third day
Week 7	Vanco, 125 mg	Once every third day
Weeks 8-11	Florastor, 250 mg	Twice per day

Note that the first week of treatment is just like what we recommend for the first or second attack: One tablet of Vanco (125 milligrams) four times per day, for a week. After that, the dose is lowered to three times per day, then twice per day, then one tablet per day. After that the Vanco is taken at a dosage of one tablet every other day, and finally for the last two weeks one tablet every third day. Florastor, a probiotic tablet that contains a harmless yeast, is added at the end of the taper to help the normal flora come back.

After this treatment plan, about 50% of patients will be cured. That is, they will no longer get watery diarrhea every hour, and there will be no more cramps, fever, etc. We know that C. diff recurrence can be delayed up to three months, so we don't declare a "cure" until the patient is having normal bowel movements beyond 90 days from the last dose of Vanco.

If the patient does get diarrhea during the 90-day, post-treatment period, the first thing we do is get a stool test to make sure it's C. diff and not some other form of diarrhea. As recounted in Chapter 1, Martina's diarrhea resulted not from recurrent infection, but from post-infectious irritable bowel syndrome. Other causes of diarrhea can also pop up after treatment including celiac disease, ulcerative colitis, Crohn's disease or even food-borne infection like Shigella, Salmonella, or Campylobacter.

You won't be able to sort this out yourself, so this situation will require an experienced doctor to order the tests and decide what to do next. The bottom line: Make sure it's C. diff and not something else causing the diarrhea.

Stool Transplant

Stool transplant, also known as a fecal transplant, is a unique therapy. At our hospital, we recommend stool transplants only if all else has failed.

Specifically, if a patient has had recurrence of C. diff, even after pulse-tapered Vanco treatment, or multiple bouts of Vanco, Dificid or Flagyl, it's time to consider a stool transplant.

The idea behind a stool transplant is to "reseed the lawn," so to speak. After exposure to weeks or months of antibiotics (including Vanco) the normal bowel flora — the organisms in your colon that help prevent infection — is weakened. They simply can't keep C. diff out. In other words, the normal barrier function of the colonic flora is gone, and C. diff gets right back in. So putting in some normal flora from a healthy donor is like reseeding the lawn — it restores the barrier. When that happens, C. diff cannot get back in, and the infection is cured.

The success rate of stool transplant is very high. We expect eventual cure in 90% or more of patients who undergo this treatment. The transplant itself is straightforward and low risk. As described in the case study involving Al the electrician, the procedure involves several steps:

1. The patient takes a laxative preparation to clean out the bowel

2. The doctor performs a colonoscopy. This involves inserting into the colon a scope, which is a thin, flexible tube that has a tiny camera and other instruments attached to the tip (see image, below).

3. When the scope reaches the top part of the colon, the doctor injects through the scope a feces suspension prepared from a healthy donor, usually a family member or close friend.

4. The scope is slowly withdrawn. As it is withdrawn, and more fecal suspension is put in from the top to bottom of the colon.

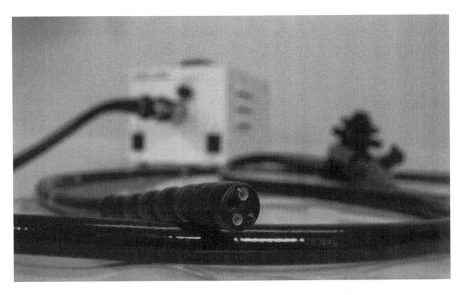

This procedure takes about 20-30 minutes, after which the patient goes home. All antibiotics are stopped the night before the procedure, to make sure that the transplanted or donor bacteria survive. Some patients feel better starting the next day, and most report no more diarrhea over the next few days. In our group of more than 30 patients transplanted over the past few years, all have been cured permanently except one (and this patient had a second stool transplant that was successful).

Some patients are too squeamish or even "grossed out" to accept this kind of treatment. It certainly seems weird to consider putting someone else's feces into your colon. But so far this approach is very safe, and the results are impressive. Thousands of such fecal transplants have been performed in the U.S. and Europe, and acceptance by both patients and doctors has been excellent.

Other Treatment Options

Some older or very ill patients may not be suitable candidates for fecal transfer. Colonoscopy is an invasive procedure, especially for those patients who are too ill with other conditions like cancer, heart failure, dialysis, or Alzheimer's. For those patients we sometimes recommend chronic Vanco therapy to suppress the C. diff and control the diarrhea.

It works like this. Vanco is a great antibiotic against C. diff. So far, C. diff has not developed resistance to Vanco. You may have heard of Vancomycin-resistant enterococcus (VRE) or Methicillin-resistant Staphylococcus Aureus (MRSA), two dangerous infections that are common in hospitals and often very hard to eradicate. But C. diff has not developed any resistance to Vanco, so as little as one tablet (125 milligrams) once daily or even every other day can be enough to keep C. diff diarrhea in check. I use this approach to manage patients with multiple C. diff recurrences who are too sick for fecal transplant, or simply refuse to have a transplant. Patients must take the Vanco indefinitely, because once it is stopped an acute attack of diarrhea will likely follow, which could be quite serious in view of their overall poor health. This treatment plan is not much different from patients with hypertension who are required to take pills to control high blood pressure for the rest of their lives.

The main downside of chronic or lifelong Vanco therapy is cost. As described earlier, Vanco is not cheap — patients without insurance coverage may have to pay up to $1,200 for 30 capsules. Not all health insurance policies cover Vanco, especially if it is going to be taken indefinitely on a daily or every other day basis.

Chapter 4:

The Future Of C. Diff

C. diff is now galloping across the globe at a rapid pace. The more antibiotics doctors prescribe, the more cases of C. diff will occur. This pathogen is very entrenched in nursing homes and hospitals, where the spores contaminate the environment. Despite our best efforts at hand washing and environmental cleansing, it is not likely that we will get rid of C. diff in health-care facilities.

In addition, cutting back on antibiotic usage is not easy. Patients with simple colds or bronchitis want their doctors to prescribe antibiotics when they are sick, even though antibiotics don't really help these viral infections. Bottom line: C. diff will continue to expand as our population ages and antibiotic usage increases.

A C. diff Vaccine?

Probably the best way to control C. diff is to develop a vaccine. We already know that vaccination of animals (rats, mice, rabbits, etc.) is highly successful in protecting them against C. diff. Also, people that carry C. diff as infants probably develop lifelong immunity that protects them from getting C. diff. Early vaccine studies in humans have been encouraging. Healthy young men when vaccinated with killed C. diff toxins (called toxoid) develop high levels of antibodies against C. diff. Studies are now underway to show that a C. diff vaccine protects patients when they are exposed to the organism in hospitals. If successful, vaccination will be made available to all, just like the vaccines used for mumps, measles, pneumonia, and influenza.

Vaccination isn't perfect because we know that vaccinated individuals can still get infected, as for example after a flu shot. But we know that vaccination can reduce both the incidence (number of cases) and severity of infections. For some diseases, such smallpox, worldwide vaccination has eradicated these awful infections from the planet. I think that vaccination will eventually help us control C. diff infection, and perhaps in time will make C. diff a distant memory.

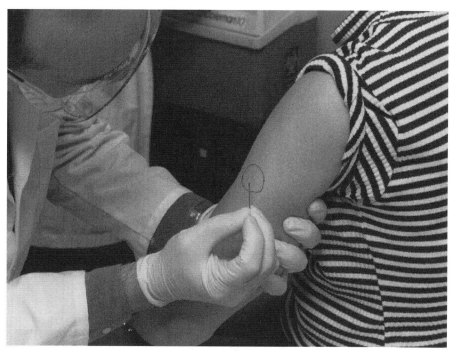

About The Author

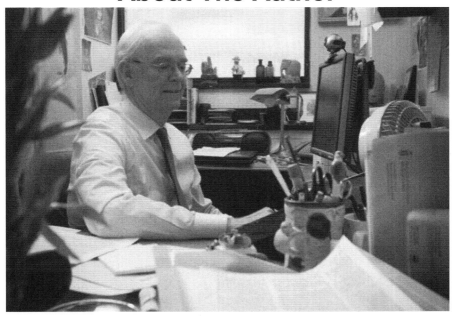

J. Thomas Lamont, M.D. received his medical degree in 1965 from the University of Rochester, and was intern, resident and chief resident in medicine at UCLA. Following a GI Fellowship at Massachusetts General Hospital, he joined the faculty of Harvard Medical School in 1974. From 1980 to 1995, he was Chief of GI at Boston University School of Medicine, and from 1996 to 2012 was GI Division Chief at Beth Israel Deaconess Medical Center. He has served as Professor of Medicine at Harvard Medical School since 1996.

Dr. Lamont's clinical interests are in the area of intestinal infections, particularly the management of C. diff infections. He and his colleagues have made a number of important discoveries about C. diff infections, including how to diagnose C. diff in patients with inflammatory bowel disease, and how the immune system protects against this infection. His group has published important papers on the C. diff carrier state, vaccine development and fecal transplant for recurrent C. diff In addition to his clinical activities, Dr. Lamont serves as a mentor for young scientists and faculty members, and as a resource for manuscript, grant preparation, and career planning. He currently serves as Associate Editor for GI and Liver Diseases at *The New England Journal of Medicine*, and as Editor-in-Chief for Gastroenterology for *UpToDate in Medicine*.

Glossary

Antibodies – Special proteins produced by immune cells that live in your spleen, lymph nodes, and other organs including the bowel. Antibodies protect you by binding to bacteria or bacterial toxins and neutralizing them so they are harmless.

Azithromycin – A type of antibiotic used to treat colds and sinusitis that is sometimes associated with C. diff infections.

Bactrim – A type of antibiotic that is sometimes associated with C. diff infections.

Biopsy – A surgical procedure to take cell or tissue samples.

C. diff (Clostridium difficile) – A serious bacterial infection of the colon (large bowel).

C. diff spore – When C. diff leaves the body, it converts to a spore that can be picked up by other people and cause a new infection. The spores can lie dormant for weeks or even months and require disinfectants like bleach or ammonia to destroy.

Cephalosporins – A class of common antibiotics that includes Keflex. It is sometimes associated with C. diff infections.

Ciprofloxacin or **Cipro** – An antibiotic that is sometimes associated with C. diff infections.

Colectomy – Surgical removal of the colon.

Colitis – Inflammation of the colon that causes diarrhea.

Colon (large intestine or **large bowel)** – The end of the digestive tract where stool is produced. Chapter 2 contains a diagram.

Colonic flora (also called **intestinal flora, bowel flora,** or **barrier flora**) – Microorganisms living in the colon that perform digestive and protective functions. Certain types of antibiotics can reduce the barrier function of the colonic flora, which in turn can lead to C. diff.

Colonoscopy – A procedure in which a long, thin, flexible tube with a camera and other instruments is inserted into the colon to examine it or gather samples. The tube can also be used to apply treatments, as is done in a stool transplant.

Culturelle (Lactobacillus GG) – A probiotic.

Dehydration – A condition caused by loss of water or other fluids in the body. Dehydration can lead to fast pulse, low blood pressure, fainting, headaches, dizziness, and even death in extreme cases.

Fidaxomycin – An antibiotic used to treat C. diff, sometimes called Fidaxo. The commercial drug name is Dificid.

Florastor – A type of probiotic used to treat C. diff. It's a yeast (S. boulardii) that is actually related to brewer's yeast, used to make beer. Florastor is freeze-dried and supplied in tablet form to be taken by mouth.

Fulminant C. diff – The most severe form of acute C. diff that sometimes affects older patients or patients with other severe medical issues. This is a serious complication and carries the risk of prolonged hospital stay, surgery, or even death.

Gastroenteritis (viral gastroenteritis) – Viral infection of the stomach and intestines. Symptoms include vomiting and diarrhea.

Ileostomy – A procedure in which patients who have had their colons removed have a permanent bag attached to their sides to catch bodily waste.

Imodium (Loperamide) – An over-the-counter anti-diarrheal pill.

Inciting Antibiotic – Antibiotics that can weaken the colonic flora and can lead to new C. diff infections.

Intensive care unit (ICU) – A hospital area for seriously ill or injured patients.

Irritable bowel syndrome (IBS) – A type of diarrhea that can follow a bowel infection like C. diff or salmonella food poisoning

Levofloxacin (levoquin) – Antibiotic associated with C. diff infections.

Lining cells – The cells that line the colon.

Metronidazole – An antibiotic used to treat C. diff. Also known as metro. Flagyl is the trade name of the drug in the U.S.

Norovirus – A very contagious virus that causes inflammation of the stomach and intestine, and symptoms such as nausea, vomiting, and diarrhea.

Post-convalescent C. diff carrier state – A patient who has C. diff and is passing C. diff spores in his or her stool, which can infect other people, but otherwise does not show diarrhea or other C. diff symptoms.

Probiotics – Dried bacteria or yeasts that are designed to help the intestinal flora, the bacteria and other microorganisms that live in our colon to return to their original state before the patient took antibiotic treatment.

Pulse-taper – A C. diff treatment that involves giving gradually smaller doses of Vanco and finally a probiotic over an 8-12-week period.

Recurrence rate – The percentage of C. diff sufferers who re-experience at least one bout of C. diff after the initial treatment.

Recurrent C. diff – When C. diff returns in a patient after an initial course of treatment.

Repeaters – Sufferers of recurrent C. diff that doesn't seem to go away.

Salmonella – A type of bacteria that causes food poisoning. Symptoms include diarrhea, abdominal cramps, and fever.

Stool – Feces or poop.

Stool transplant (fecal transplant) - A procedure in which fecal matter from a healthy person is transplanted to the colon of a patient suffering from recurrent C. diff.

Sub-total colectomy – Surgery to remove part of the colon

Toxic megacolon – Seriously infected and dilated lower bowel caused by infections including C. diff.

Toxin A and **Toxin B** – Released by C. diff bacteria into the colon, these toxins cause inflammation and diarrhea in patients.

Treating Antibiotics – Antibiotics such as Flagyl, Vanco, and Dificid that are often used to treat C. diff.

Vancomycin (Vanco) – An antibiotic used to treat C. diff. Vancocin or Vanco is the commercial version of the drug.

Online Resources

Here are some reliable health information sites for patients interested in learning more about C. diff:

Mayo Clinic (mayoclinic.com): C. difficile

Centers for Disease Control and Prevention (cdc.gov/hai): Clostridium difficile Infection

National Institutes of Health/MedLine Plus (www.nlm.nih.gov/medlineplus): Clostridium Difficile Infections

Note that there are many other web sites and online forums that discuss C. diff and various treatments. Be very careful about the recommendations and advice published on such sites. While some people have useful experiences to share about dealing with C. diff, others may be promoting untested, bogus, or even harmful treatments. If you are diagnosed with C. diff, consult with your doctor about recommended treatment options.

Image Credits

Chapter 2: Scanning electron micrograph of Escherichia coli, grown in culture and adhered to a cover slip. Credit: Rocky Mountain Laboratories, NIAID, NIH. Source: National Institutes of Health.

Chapter 4: A doctor uses a two-pronged needle to deliver the smallpox vaccine into the arm of a volunteer in a smallpox vaccination dilution study. Credit: University of Rochester School of Medicine.

Stock photographs of people, as well as the graphic showing the location of the colon (Chapter 2) were licensed from Shutterstock.

All other photographs, images, tables, and diagrams were created by i30 Media.

More In 30 Minutes® Guides

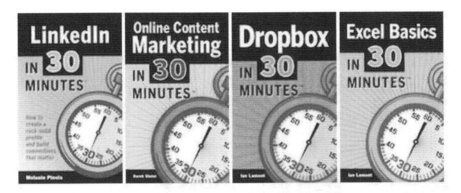

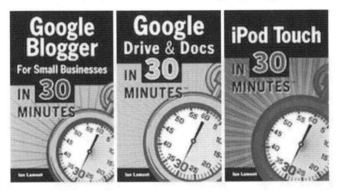

In 30 Minutes® guides can help you get started with LinkedIn, Google Drive, Dropbox, and other topics. The guides are written in plain English, with lots of step-by-step instructions and practical advice. Here's what real readers are saying:

Dropbox In 30 Minutes:

> "This was truly a 30-minute tutorial and I have mastered the basics without bugging my 20-year-old son! Yahoo!"

Google Drive & Docs In 30 Minutes:

"I've been using Google Docs for a while now and have been encouraging my teacher colleagues to do so as well to facilitate collaboration. It has become my go-to text book to help new users understand quickly. If you're new to Google Drive or Google Documents, this will help you."

Excel Basics In 30 Minutes:

"I have used Excel in the past in only a very limited fashion. I learned from your book how to use formulas, make charts, and sort. I will have to play with the charts a little more - there are so many options that it feels like a whole other program! The "ninja" autofill function is awesome!"

All guides are available as paperbacks and in ebook formats, including downloads for the Kindle, iPad, and Nook. They can also be downloaded as full-color PDFs. Visit In30Minutes.com to learn more about the guides, and access purchase links, free videos, blog posts, and other resources!

Made in the USA
San Bernardino, CA
07 February 2014